Autoimmune Paleo Cookbook

The Complete Paleo Food List

30 Easy and Quick Autoimmune Paleo Recipes

BY

Rachael Rayner

Copyright 2016 Rachael Rayner

License Notes

No part of this Book can be reproduced in any form or by any means including print, electronic, scanning or photocopying unless prior permission is granted by the author.

All ideas, suggestions and guidelines mentioned here are written for informative purposes. While the author has taken every possible step to ensure accuracy, all readers are advised to follow information at their own risk. The author cannot be held responsible for personal and/or commercial damages in case of misinterpreting and misunderstanding any part of this Book

Table of Contents

Introduction

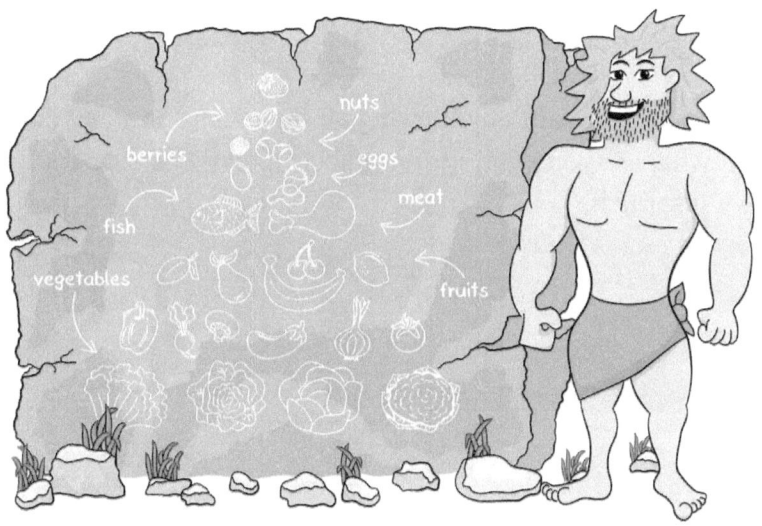

A Palaeolithic diet is an ancient diet that is all about eating fresh fruit, vegetables, eggs, meat, chicken, nuts and fish and cutting down dairy products, sugar, grains and potatoes and processed foods.

This cookbook you will help you out in making easy and quick traditional and contemporary paleo autoimmune recipes that can be used for breakfast, lunch, dinner, or brunch for any occasion or get together.

It contains an extensive collection of delectable and seductive paleo autoimmune dishes that will make you look, and feel healthier. Each recipe has easy to follow steps as well as a picture to allow you to see what the finished product will look like.

I am sure you will enjoy trying all the recipes in this book. So what are you waiting for, grab your copy now and let's get it started!

Shrimp Salad with Mint Dressing

Very refreshing and healthy salad recipe that can be enjoyed in lunch or snack time.

Preparation time: 25 minutes

Yield: 3 servings

Ingredients:

- 1 oz. shrimps
- 2 tablespoons olive oil
- 2 tablespoons lemon juice
- 2-3 garlic cloves, minced
- ½ teaspoon black pepper
- ¼ teaspoon salt
- 1 green chili
- 2 avocadoes, pitted, chopped
- 1 bunch kale leaves, chopped
- 2 carrots, shredded
- 1 cup coconut milk
- 1 bunch mint leaves

Method:

1. In a blender add coconut milk, green chill, lemon juice and mint leaves, blend well.

2. Heat oil in saucepan and sauté shrimps for 5 minutes.

3. Season with salt and pepper.

4. Turn off heat and transfer into serving dish with carrots, avocado and kale.

5. Serve salad with mint dressing and enjoy.

Cucumber and Avocado Dill Smoothie

If you are looking for delicious and healthy smoothie then this is perfect for you.

Preparation time: 5 minutes

Yield: 2 servings

Ingredients:

- 1 cucumber, peeled, sliced
- 2 tablespoons dill, chopped
- 2 tablespoons lemon juice
- 1 avocado, pitted
- 1 cup coconut milk
- 1 teaspoon coconut, shredded
- 2 kiwis, peeled, sliced

Method:

1. In a blender add all ingredients and blend well.

2. Drain the extract and discard residue.

3. Serve and enjoy.

Grilled Beef with Pineapple Marinade

Mouth-melting and sizzling marinade recipe, it will blow you mind.

Preparation time: 25 minutes

Yield: 4 servings

Ingredients:

- 2 oz. beef steaks
- 2 tablespoons lemon juice
- 1 cup pineapple juice
- ½ cup pineapple
- 1 teaspoon sea salt
- 1 teaspoon garlic paste
- 1 teaspoon ginger paste
- 2 tablespoons coconut oil

Method:

1. In a blender add pineapple, oil, lemon juice, pineapple juice, salt, ginger garlic paste and blend well.

2. Pour this mixture on steaks and rub with hands.

3. Cover and place into fridge for 10-15 minutes.

4. Preheat grill and grease with oil.

5. Now place steaks on heated grill, leave to cook until nicely brown from both sides.

6. Serve and enjoy.

Healthy Bone Broth

This highly nutritious delight is made with just few and simple ingredient.

Preparation time: 2 hours

Yield: 5 servings

Ingredients:

- 1 oz. bones, cleaned
- 2 tablespoons apple cider vinegar
- 1 onion, sliced
- 5-6 garlic cloves
- 1 tablespoon cooking oil
- ½ teaspoon salt
- ½ teaspoon white pepper
- 1 inch ginger slice
- 5 cups water

Method:

1. In large skillet add bones with water, onion, garlic, ginger, oil, vinegar, salt, pepper and stir. Cover with lid.

2. Leave to cook on low heat for 2 hours.

3. Strain the broth and discard residue.

4. Serve hot and enjoy.

Stir Fried Chicken with Cabbage

This fresh looking dish is made with chicken and shredded cabbage and seasoned with salt and pepper.

Preparation time: 25 minutes

Yield: 4 servings

Ingredients:

- 1 oz. chicken, boneless, small pieces
- 1 cup cabbage, shredded
- ½ teaspoon garlic paste
- ¼ teaspoon ginger paste
- ¼ teaspoon salt
- ½ teaspoon black pepper
- 2 tablespoons lemon juice
- 2 tablespoons coconut oil

Method:

1. Heat oil in pan and sauté garlic for 1 minute.

2. Add chicken and fry till nicely brown.

3. Add cabbage and stir for 5-10 minutes.

4. Season with salt and pepper.

5. Add lemon juice and turn off heat.

6. Serve and enjoy.

Strawberry and Cherry Shake

This shake is absolutely a great boost with wonderful taste.

Preparation time: 5 minutes

Yield: 2 servings

Ingredients:

- 1 cup strawberries
- 1 cup cherries
- 1 cup almond milk
- ½ cup coconut milk
- 2 tablespoons brown sugar
- Few ice chunks

Method:

1. In a blender add all ingredients and blend well.

2. Serve and enjoy.

Chicken Mince with Peas

A traditional chicken mince recipe with peas that are cooking in tomato puree.

Preparation time: 35 minutes

Yield: 4 servings

Ingredients:

- 1 oz. minced chicken
- 1 onion, chopped
- 1 cup peas
- 1 cup tomato puree
- ¼ teaspoon garlic paste
- ½ teaspoon chili powder
- ¼ teaspoon turmeric powder
- 1 bunch fresh coriander, chopped
- 1 lemon
- 2 green chilies
- ½ teaspoon cumin powder
- ½ teaspoon cinnamon powder
- 2 cups chicken broth
- ¼ teaspoon salt
- 2 tablespoons olive oil

Method:

1. Heat oil in pan and add onion, fry for 2 minute.

2. Add chicken mince with garlic and fry well till nicely golden.

3. Add tomato puree and fry again for 5-10 minutes.

4. Add salt, chili powder, turmeric powder. Stir.

5. Add peas and fry for 5 minutes.

6. Transfer chicken broth and cover with lid. Leave to cook on low heat for 15 minutes.

7. Sprinkle cumin and cinnamon powder.

8. Transfer into serving dish and top with coriander and green chilies.

9. Squeeze lemon juice.

10. Serve and enjoy.

Chicken Minced Stuffed Bell Peppers

These flavourful stuffed bell peppers are very yummy to eat.

Preparation time: 35 minutes

Yield: 4 servings

Ingredients:

- 2 red bell peppers, make a cut from stem
- 2 yellow bell peppers, make a cut from stem
- 1 cup chicken mince
- ½ cup tomato puree
- ¼ teaspoon garlic paste
- ½ teaspoon black pepper
- ¼ teaspoon salt
- 2 tablespoons olive oil

Method:

1. Heat oil in pan and add garlic, fry for 1 minute.

2. Add chicken mince and stir well.

3. When chicken mince become golden brown add tomato puree and fry again for 5-10 minutes.

4. Season with salt and pepper.

5. Preheat oven at 355 degrees.

6. Fill bell peppers with fried mince and place into greased pan.

7. Bake for 10 minutes.

8. Serve and enjoy.

Stir Fried Zucchini with Ground Beef

This recipe is very easy and delicious to taste.

Preparation time: 25 minutes

Yield: 3 servings

Ingredients:

- 1 oz. beef mince
- 2 zucchinis, sliced
- 1 onion, sliced
- ½ teaspoon garlic paste
- ½ teaspoons ground cumin seeds
- ¼ teaspoons cumin powder
- 2 tablespoons vinegar
- ½ cup chicken broth
- ¼ teaspoon salt
- ¼ teaspoon chili powder
- 2 tablespoons coconut oil

Method:

1. Heat oil in pan and sauté garlic with onion for 1 minute.

2. Add beef mince and fry till nicely brown.

3. Add zucchini and stir well.

4. Fry for 5 minutes on medium heat.

5. Add in chicken broth, salt, chili powder, vinegar, leave to cook on low heat for 10-15 minutes.

6. When water is dried out add cumin and cinnamon powder. Stir well.

7. Serve and enjoy.

Fresh Pomegranate Brew

Make this delicious drink and forget all other expensive and unhealthy drinks.

Preparation time: 10 minutes

Yield: 2 servings

Ingredients:

- 2 cups pomegranate seeds
- 1 inch ginger slice
- 2 mint leaves
- 1 cup ice chunks
- ½ cup cherry juice
- 1 tablespoons brown sugar

Method:

1. In blend add all ingredients and blend well.

2. Strain juice and remove remaining.

3. Add to serving glass and serve.

Grapefruit and Radish Salad

This colourful salad is very healthy for any abdominal disease.

Preparation time: 10 minutes

Yield: 3 servings

Ingredients:

- 1 cup grapefruit flashes, peeled
- 1 radish, sliced
- 1 cup cabbage, chopped
- ½ cup pineapple juice
- 1 pinch of salt
- 2 tablespoons apple cider vinegar
- 1 teaspoon fresh dill, chopped

Method:

1. In a medium bowl add pineapple juice, vinegar, salt, and mix.

2. Now add cabbage, radish, and grapefruit, toss to combine well.

3. Sprinkle dill on top.

4. Serve and enjoy.

Ginger Zest Watermelon Shrub

This juice is very effective for inflammation.

Preparation time: 10 minutes

Yield: 2 servings

Ingredients:

- 2 cups watermelon chunks, seeded
- 2 tablespoons lemon juice
- 1 inch ginger slice
- 1 cup water
- 1 cup ice chunks

Method:

1. Take a juicer and add watermelon chunks, lemon juice, ginger slice, ice and water. Blend till puree.

2. Add to serving glasses and serve.

Cooling Fruit Bowl

This is so much yummy and lively bowl that is filled with easily available fruits.

Preparation time: 10 minutes

Yield: 3 servings

Ingredients:

- 2 bananas, sliced
- 2 tablespoons lemon juice
- 1 cup strawberries, halved
- 1 cup grapes
- 2 oranges, peeled
- 1 cup pineapple, chunks

Method:

1. In a bowl add all fruits and toss to combine.

2. Drizzle lemon juice on top and serve.

Spinach Curry

This delight is simple made with blended spinach and cooked with the flavours of ginger and garlic.

Preparation time: 30 minutes

Yield: 5 servings

Ingredients:

- 2 cups spinach leaves, chopped
- 2 cups chicken broth
- 1 teaspoon garlic paste
- 2 inch ginger slice, shredded
- ¼ teaspoon turmeric powder
- ¼ teaspoon salt
- 1 green chili
- 1 tablespoon coconut oil
- ½ cup water

Method:

1. In a blender add spinach with water and green chili, blend till puree.

2. Now heat oil in pan and add ginger with garlic, sauté for 1 minute.

3. Add spinach and fry for 5 minutes or its colour is slightly changed.

4. Pour chicken broth and add salt, leave to cook on low heat for 15-20 minutes.

5. Serve and enjoy.

Chicken Roast

This chicken roasted is made with rosemary, orange juice and ginger marinade and delicious to eat.

Preparation time: 40 minutes

Yield: 6 servings

Ingredients:

- 1 whole chicken
- 2 tablespoons lemon juice
- 3 tablespoons vinegar
- 1 tablespoon dried rosemary
- ½ cup orange juice
- ½ teaspoon ginger paste
- ½ teaspoon garlic paste
- ½ teaspoon salt
- 2 tablespoons fish sauce
- ½ teaspoon black pepper
- ¼ teaspoon sea salt
- ½ teaspoon cinnamon powder
- 2 tablespoons olive oil

Method:

1. Preheat oven at 355 degrees.

2. In a bowl add orange juice, rosemary, oil, lemon juice, vinegar, ginger garlic paste, fish sauce, salt, pepper, rosemary and mix well.

3. Rub this mixture on chicken thoroughly.

4. Place chicken into a greased pan and bake for 30-35 minutes or until golden brown.

Coconut Milk Banana Cocktail

This is highly scrumptious cocktail recipe that can be made in just few minutes.

Preparation time: 5 minutes

Yield: 1 servings

Ingredients:

- 1 cup coconut milk
- 2 ripe bananas
- 2 tablespoons brown sugar
- ¼ teaspoon cardamom powder
- 6-7 ice cubes

Method:

1. In blender add coconut milk with cardamom powder, brown sugar, bananas and blend well.

2. Pour into glass and add ice chunks.

3. Serve and enjoy.

Beef Stew with Fried Mushrooms

This is traditional stew recipe with the taste of mushrooms.

Preparation time: 1 hour 15 minutes

Yield: 3 servings

Ingredients:

- 1 oz. beef meat
- 4-5 garlic cloves, minced
- 4 cups water
- 1 onion, sliced
- 3 tablespoons oil
- ½ teaspoon black pepper
- 1 bay leaf
- 1 clove
- ¼ teaspoon cumin powder
- 1 cup mushrooms, sliced

Method:

1. Heat oil in a skillet and add mushrooms, fry for 5 minutes and place aside.

2. In the same skillet add onion and sauté with bay leaf and clove for 1-2 minutes.

3. Now add beef and garlic, fry well till its colour become brownish.

4. Add water and leave to cook on low heat for 1 hour.

5. Now transfer fried mushrooms, salt, pepper, cumin powder and stir well.

6. Discard bay leaf.

7. Turn off heat after 10 minutes.

8. Serve hot and enjoy.

Yummy Lamb Hash

This cousin is loaded with flavours and nutrition. Your family will love this hash.

Preparation time: 10 minutes

Yield: 3 servings

Ingredients:

- 1 oz. lamb meat, boiled
- 1 cup tomato puree
- 1 onion, sliced
- 3-4 garlic cloves
- 1 cup vegetable broth
- 2 tablespoons vinegar
- 2 tablespoons olive oil
- 1 teaspoon chili powder
- ½ teaspoon salt
- ¼ teaspoon turmeric powder
- ½ teaspoon cumin powder
- ½ teaspoon cinnamon powder

Method:

1. Heat oil in pan and add onion, cook until lightly golden.

2. Now add boiled lamb and fry for 10 minutes.

3. Add tomato puree, salt, chili powder, turmeric powder, vinegar and fry for 5 minutes on high heat.

4. Add vegetable broth and leave to cook on low heat for 15 minutes.

5. Now sprinkle cumin powder, cinnamon powder and turn off heat.

6. Serve and enjoy.

Paleo Pancakes

These scrumptious pancakes are gluten and lactose free.

Preparation time: 10 minutes

Yield: 4 servings

Ingredients:

- 2 eggs
- 4 tablespoons almond flour
- ½ cup coconut, shredded
- 2 bananas
- 1 pinch salt
- 2 tablespoons brown sugar
- ¼ cup coconut milk
- 2 tablespoons coconut oil

Method:

1. In a bowl add bananas and mash with folk.

2. Crack eggs in it and whisk well.

3. Add flour, salt, brown sugar, milk, coconut and mix thoroughly.

4. Heat oil in non-stick pan and pour 4-5 tablespoons of batter, spread in the form of cake and leave to cook until nicely brown from both sides.

5. Enjoy.

Grilled Salmon

This dish is bursting with flavours that will blow your mind.

Preparation time: 35

Yield: 2 servings

Ingredients:

- 2 salmon fillets
- ½ teaspoon garlic paste
- 3 tablespoons lemon juice
- 1 teaspoon salt
- ½ teaspoon black pepper
- ½ teaspoon oregano
- 1 teaspoon fish sauce
- ¼ teaspoon turmeric powder
- 2 tablespoons olive oil

Method:

1. Sprinkle turmeric powder on fish and rub all over.

2. Leave it for 10-15 minutes then wash out fish well.

3. Take a bowl add vinegar, lemon juice, pepper, salt, fish sauce and oregano, toss to combine.

4. Spread this mixture on fish fillets and rub on it with hands.

5. Preheat grill and spray with oil.

6. Place fish fillets on grill and let to brown well.

7. Flip the side and make sure both sides are cooked well.

8. Serve and enjoy.

Carrots and Broccoli Stew

Very tendered and tongue tingling carrots and broccoli dish.

Preparation time: 45

Yield: 4 servings

Ingredients:

- 2 carrots, peppered, sliced
- 1 cup broccoli florets
- 3 cup chicken broth
- 1 cup water
- 1 onion, sliced
- 2-3 garlic cloves, minced
- 1 teaspoon salt
- ½ teaspoon black pepper
- 2 tablespoons olive oil

Method:

1. Heat oil in a skillet and sauté onion for 1-2 minutes.

2. Add garlic and stir for 30 seconds.

3. Now add carrots and broccoli, sauté for 5-10 minutes on medium heat.

4. Now add water, chicken broth, salt, pepper and stir.

5. Cover with lid and leave to cook on low heat for 25-30 minutes.

6. Serve and enjoy.

Traditional Poached Eggs in Tomato Sauce

This delight is made with eggs that are cooked in tomato curry, it is perfect dish for breakfast.

Preparation time: 35

Yield: 4 servings

Ingredients:

- 4 eggs
- 1 onion, sliced
- 1 onion, chopped
- 1 cup tomato puree
- 1 cup tomato sauce
- 1 teaspoon salt
- ½ teaspoon black pepper
- 2 tablespoons olive oil

Method:

1. Heat oil in a pan and sauté onion for 1-2 minutes.

2. Add tomato puree, tomato sauce and fry for 10-15 minutes.

3. Now make four small wells in the tomato gravy and crack egg into each well.

4. Cover with lid and leave to cook on low heat for 10 minutes.

5. Sprinkle salt and pepper on top.

6. Serve and enjoy.

Cucumber Salad with Tomatoes and Onion

Cucumber and tomatoes are very effective to improve immune system.

Preparation time: 5 minutes

Yield: 2 servings

Ingredients:

- 1 cucumber, peeled, chopped
- 1 onion, sliced
- 2 tomatoes, chopped
- ¼ teaspoon salt
- ¼ teaspoon black pepper
- ¼ teaspoon cinnamon powder
- 2 tablespoons apple cider vinegar
- 2 tablespoons lemon juice

Method:

1. In a bowl add ingredients and toss to combine.

2. Transfer into serving dish.

3. Serve and enjoy.

Paleo Egg Curry

This is traditional and classical egg recipe that can be enjoyed in breakfast of lunch.

Preparation time: 35

Yield: 3 servings

Ingredients:

- 2 eggs, hard boiled, halved
- 1 onion, sliced
- 1 onion, chopped
- 1 cup tomato puree
- 1 teaspoon salt
- ½ teaspoon black pepper
- ½ teaspoon cumin powder
- ¼ teaspoon cinnamon powder
- 2 tablespoons olive oil
- ¼ cup water

Method:

1. Heat oil in a pan and sauté onion for 1-2 minutes.

2. Add tomato puree and fry for 10-15 minutes.

3. Now add water and leave to cook for 5-10 minutes.

4. When water is dried out add salt, pepper, cumin powder, cinnamon powder and mix well.

5. Add eggs and toss to combine.

6. Turn off heat and serve hot.

7. Serve and enjoy.

Paleo Styled Egg Salad

This salad recipe is very simple, easy to make and an absolute taste.

Preparation time: 15

Yield: 3 servings

Ingredients:

- 3 eggs, boiled, sliced
- 2 tomatoes, chopped
- 1 cup cabbages, chopped
- 1 cup broccoli florets
- 1 carrot, sliced
- 2-3 lettuce leaves, sliced
- 1 teaspoon salt
- ½ teaspoon black pepper

Method:

1. Take a large bowl and add tomatoes, broccoli, carrot slices, lettuce and cabbage, toss to combine.

2. Place egg slices and season with salt and pepper.

3. Enjoy.

Grapefruit and Orange Extract

This juice is made with grapefruit, orange, lemon juice, ginger and brown sugar.

Preparation time: 5

Yield: 2 servings

Ingredients:

- 1 cup grapefruit, peeled, flashes
- 3 oranges, peeled
- 1 inch ginger slice
- 2 tablespoons brown sugar
- 1 cup crushed ice

Method:

1. In a blender add all ingredients and blend till puree.

2. Now strain the extract and discard the residue.

3. Pour to serving glasses and serve immediately.

Paleo Carrot Salad

This salad is made with grated carrots and freshly chopped dill and lemon juice.

Preparation time: 5

Yield: 2 servings

Ingredients:

- 3 carrots, peeled, grated
- 2 tablespoons lemon juice
- 1 tablespoon chopped dill
- 1 tablespoons vinegar

Method:

1. In a platter add carrots, drizzle lemon juice and vinegar, toss to combine.

2. Now sprinkle dill on top and serve.

3. Enjoy.

Paleo Minty Watermelon Salad

This is highly refreshing salad recipe that can be done in snap.

Preparation time: 15

Yield: 2 servings

Ingredients:

- 1 watermelon
- 2 tablespoons lemon juice
- 2 tablespoons brown sugar
- 1 tablespoons freshly chopped mint leaves
- ½ cup orange juice

Method:

1. In bowl add orange juice, brown sugar, lemon juice, mint leave and mix well.

2. Scoop out watermelon and add to serving bowl, pour orange juice mixture on top and serve.

3. Enjoy.

Pineapple and Kiwi Lime Salad

This salad is made with pineapple, kiwi, bananas, strawberry and orange with the flavour or mustard and lime.

Preparation time: 5

Yield: 3 servings

Ingredients:

- 1 cup pineapple chunks
- 2 bananas, sliced
- 1/2cup strawberries, sliced
- 2 kiwis, sliced
- 1 orange, peeled
- ¼ teaspoon Dijon mustard powder
- 2-3 mint leaves chopped
- 2 tablespoons lime juice
- ½ cup pineapple juice

Method:

1. In bowl add all fruits and toss to combine.

2. Take a bowl and add lime juice, pineapple juice, mint leaves, mustard powder and mix well.

3. Pour this mixture over the fruits and toss.

4. Enjoy.

Funnel and Asparagus Salsa

This salsa it the mixture of ribboned asparagus and sliced funnel.

Preparation time: 15

Yield: 3 servings

Ingredients:

- 1 oz. asparagus, cut into ribbons
- 2 funnel bulbs, sliced
- ¼ teaspoon Dijon mustard powder
- 2 tablespoons lime juice
- 1 tablespoons freshly chopped dill

Method:

1. In bowl add ingredients and toss to combine.

2. Serve and enjoy.

Paleo Spinach Green Smoothie

This smoothie will definitely blow your mind by its taste and freshness.

Preparation time: 5

Yield: 2 servings

Ingredients:

- 1 cup baby spinach leaves
- 2-3 mint leave
- 1 cup grapes juice
- 1 cup pineapple juice
- 2 tablespoons lime juice

Method:

1. In blender add ingredients and blend well till puree.

2. Transfer to serving glasses.

3. Serve and enjoy.

Author's Afterthoughts

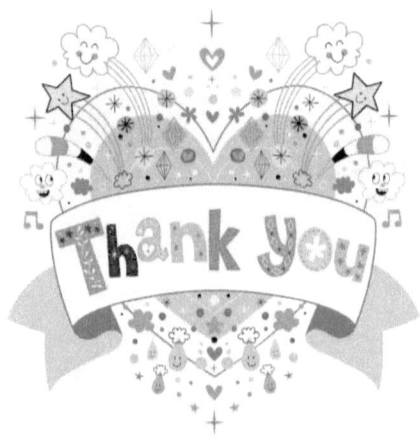

Thanks ever so much to each of my cherished readers for investing the time to read this book!

I know you could have picked from many other books but you chose this one. So a big thanks for downloading this book and reading all the way to the end.

If you enjoyed this book or received value from it, I'd like to ask you for a favor. Please take a few minutes to post an honest and heartfelt review on Amazon.com. Your support does make a difference and helps to benefit other people.

Thanks for your Reviews!

Rachael Rayner

www.ingramcontent.com/pod-product-compliance
Lightning Source LLC
Chambersburg PA
CBHW020904310526
45786CB00018B/1739